FOOD
SYMPTOM DIARY

The content of this book does not replace nutritional advice nor medical advice. The food-symptom-diary may be used for general information and structured logging of symptoms that may be associated with various foods.

In case of unexplained symptoms, prior to starting your symptom logbook medical or nutritional advice should be sought if this has not already been done.

FOOD
SYMPTOM DIARY

Logbook for symptoms with IBS, food allergies, food intolerances, indigestion, Crohn's disease, ulcerative colitis and leaky gut

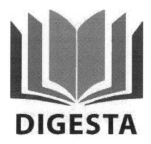

DIGESTA

Disclaimer: This booklet is not intended to provide medical advice or to replace medical advice. The book is intended to
provide helpful information on food intolerances. All readers are advised to consult a doctor/physician or other qualified
healthcare provider regarding the diagnosis or treatment of medical conditions. The understanding of this book is that the
author is neither involved in personal professional service nor engaged in rendering medical services. The author disclaims
all responsibility for any loss, liability or risk that is incurred as a direct or indirect consequence of the use and application
of any of the contents of this book. The content of this book resembles the opinion of the author and was not evaluated
by any national or international authority.

ISBN-13: 978-1545487181

ISBN-10: 1545487189

Table of contents

Introduction/ Application notes

Many abdominal symptoms related like abdominal pain, abdominal cramps, diarrhea and constipation as well as non-intestinal complaints such as headaches, dizziness, rashes, runny or blocked nose, fatigue, lightheadedness, watery eyes and other symptoms can be attributed to the diet or individual foods.

The identification of food related symptoms is usually difficult since we consume various foods during the course of a day.

Dieticians, medical practitioners and professional societies recommend using a professional food-symptom diary that logs food intake, amounts consumed and type of preparation as well as symptoms, symptom intensity and type of bowel movements (diarrhea, soft, normal, hard, none).
Such a log helps you to determine individual intolerances to foods or food ingredients.

An intolerance is likely when foods are correlated to symptoms on a regular basis, an irregular occurrence makes such a relation unlikely

In separate tables in the second part of this booklet you may list foods that are well-tolerated, foods that cause symptoms and foods that are alternately well or badly tolerated. These tables will serve as your memory of individual food tolerances and food intolerances.

The diary is kept small in size to allow you to carry it with you wherever you go. It is important that your diary accompanies you all the time to allow you to log all important information whenever food intake or symptoms happen.

In the back of this book, you'll find additional tables listing foods that are frequently, but not always, badly. These lists will help you to identify intolerances against the most frequent lead substances.

The lists include tables to identify intolerances against

Lactose
Fructose
Sorbitol
Trehalose
Fructans / Fructooligosaccharides
Galactans / Galactooligosaccharides
Gluten
Histamine
Salicylates
Biogenic Amines
Pseudoallergens (Mast Cells)

If you suspect an intolerance against one of these lead substances, you can narrow this down with the suggested test-foods.

After logging your individual intolerances for 6-8 weeks it may be helpful to discuss these records and the consequences with a doctor or dietician trained to identify the patterns behind foods causing symptoms.

For comments or suggestions, please contact the Digesta-Team (digesta@gmx.net) by e-mail.

Bristol stool scale (BSS)

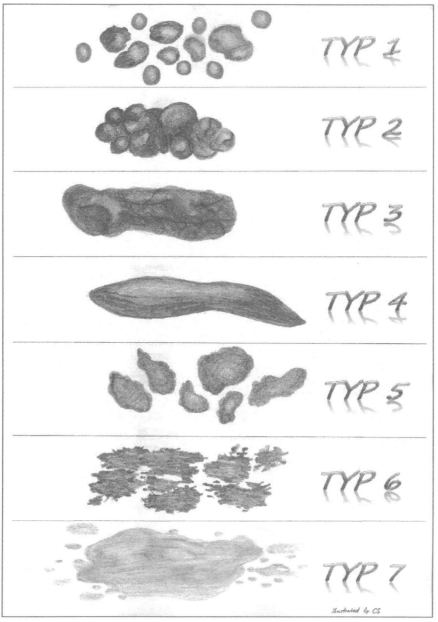

The BSS will help you to chart your bowel movements.

Type 1: separate hard lumps

Type 3: sausage like, surface cracks

Type 5: soft blobs, clear cut edges

Type 7: liquid

Type 2: lumpy, sausage like

Type 4: soft, smooth sausage

Type 6: mushy with ragged edges

time	Foods, drinks & sweets incl. amount, preparation (raw, steamed, boiled, fried, grilled, rewarmed, peeled), spices and for convenience food ingredients. Medications, vitamin supplements, food supplements, probiotics.	Symptoms	
		type, time, duration, intensity from 0 (none) – 10 (very severe), bowel movement	
			intensity
6:45	black tea with milk (200 ml)		0
7:00	yoghurt 150 g (brand name) + 1 teaspoon strawberry yam (brand name)	7:45 bowel movement (soft, type 4)	3
	bread (whole-grain) 1 slice		0
	salami 25 g (brand name)		0
11:15	chewing gum (brand name, contains sorbitol and isomaltol) 3 pieces		
12:30		bloating/gas	9
13:00	carrots, steamed (200 g)		0
16:10	probiotic (brand name) 2 capsules		0
16:15	tomato (~ 100g) - mozzarella (~ 100g)	no problems	0
18:00	beer (brand name) (dark, ½ L)	cramps	8
19:45		diarrhea (watery, type 7)	7
19:55	cucumber, peeled (100 g)		0

foods causing symptoms		
food	symptoms	bowel movement
beer (brand name)	cramps	Diarrhea (type 7)
chewing gum (Sorbitol?)	bloating/gas	

Other: activities, sport, stress, animal contact, smoking, other stress factors

Yoga from 3 - 4 pm

Date: _____   Food-Symptom-Diary

time	Foods, drinks & sweets incl. amount, preparation (raw, steamed, boiled, fried, grilled, rewarmed, peeled), spices and for convenience food ingredients. Medications, vitamin supplements, food supplements, probiotics.	Symptoms	
		type, time, duration, intensity from 0 (none) – 10 (very severe), bowel movement	
			intensity

foods causing symptoms		
food	symptoms	bowel movement

Other: activities, sport, stress, animal contact, smoking, other stress factors

Date: _____   Food-Symptom-Diary

time	Foods, drinks & sweets incl. amount, preparation (raw, steamed, boiled, fried, grilled, rewarmed, peeled), spices and for convenience food ingredients. Medications, vitamin supplements, food supplements, probiotics.	Symptoms	
		type, time, duration, intensity from 0 (none) – 10 (very severe), bowel movement	intensity

foods causing symptoms		
food	symptoms	bowel movement

Other: activities, sport, stress, animal contact, smoking, other stress factors

Date: _____   Food-Symptom-Diary

time	Foods, drinks & sweets incl. amount, preparation (raw, steamed, boiled, fried, grilled, rewarmed, peeled), spices and for convenience food ingredients. Medications, vitamin supplements, food supplements, probiotics.	Symptoms	
		type, time, duration, intensity from 0 (none) – 10 (very severe), bowel movement	intensity

foods causing symptoms		
food	symptoms	bowel movement

Other: activities, sport, stress, animal contact, smoking, other stress factors

Date: _____   Food-Symptom-Diary

time	Foods, drinks & sweets incl. amount, preparation (raw, steamed, boiled, fried, grilled, rewarmed, peeled), spices and for convenience food ingredients. Medications, vitamin supplements, food supplements, probiotics.	Symptoms	
		type, time, duration, intensity from 0 (none) – 10 (very severe), bowel movement	
			intensity

foods causing symptoms		
food	symptoms	bowel movement

Other: activities, sport, stress, animal contact, smoking, other stress factors

Date: _____   Food-Symptom-Diary

time	Foods, drinks & sweets incl. amount, preparation (raw, steamed, boiled, fried, grilled, rewarmed, peeled), spices and for convenience food ingredients. Medications, vitamin supplements, food supplements, probiotics.	Symptoms	
		type, time, duration, intensity from 0 (none) – 10 (very severe), bowel movement	intensity

foods causing symptoms		
food	symptoms	bowel movement

Other: activities, sport, stress, animal contact, smoking, other stress factors

Date: _____   Food-Symptom-Diary

time	Foods, drinks & sweets incl. amount, preparation (raw, steamed, boiled, fried, grilled, rewarmed, peeled), spices and for convenience food ingredients. Medications, vitamin supplements, food supplements, probiotics.	Symptoms	
		type, time, duration, intensity from 0 (none) – 10 (very severe), bowel movement	
			intensity

foods causing symptoms		
food	symptoms	bowel movement

Other: activities, sport, stress, animal contact, smoking, other stress factors

Date: _____   Food-Symptom-Diary

time	Foods, drinks & sweets incl. amount, preparation (raw, steamed, boiled, fried, grilled, rewarmed, peeled), spices and for convenience food ingredients. Medications, vitamin supplements, food supplements, probiotics.	Symptoms	
		type, time, duration, intensity from 0 (none) – 10 (very severe), bowel movement	intensity

foods causing symptoms		
food	symptoms	bowel movement

Other: activities, sport, stress, animal contact, smoking, other stress factors

Date: _____   Food-Symptom-Diary

time	Foods, drinks & sweets incl. amount, preparation (raw, steamed, boiled, fried, grilled, rewarmed, peeled), spices and for convenience food ingredients. Medications, vitamin supplements, food supplements, probiotics.	Symptoms	
		type, time, duration, intensity from 0 (none) – 10 (very severe), bowel movement	intensity

foods causing symptoms		
food	symptoms	bowel movement

Other: activities, sport, stress, animal contact, smoking, other stress factors

Date: _____   Food-Symptom-Diary

time	Foods, drinks & sweets incl. amount, preparation (raw, steamed, boiled, fried, grilled, rewarmed, peeled), spices and for convenience food ingredients. Medications, vitamin supplements, food supplements, probiotics.	Symptoms	
		type, time, duration, intensity from 0 (none) – 10 (very severe), bowel movement	
			intensity

foods causing symptoms		
food	symptoms	bowel movement

Other: activities, sport, stress, animal contact, smoking, other stress factors

Date: _____   Food-Symptom-Diary

time	Foods, drinks & sweets incl. amount, preparation (raw, steamed, boiled, fried, grilled, rewarmed, peeled), spices and for convenience food ingredients. Medications, vitamin supplements, food supplements, probiotics.	Symptoms	
		type, time, duration, intensity from 0 (none) – 10 (very severe), bowel movement	
			intensity

foods causing symptoms		
food	symptoms	bowel movement

Other: activities, sport, stress, animal contact, smoking, other stress factors

Date: _____   Food-Symptom-Diary

time	Foods, drinks & sweets incl. amount, preparation (raw, steamed, boiled, fried, grilled, rewarmed, peeled), spices and for convenience food ingredients. Medications, vitamin supplements, food supplements, probiotics.	Symptoms	
		type, time, duration, intensity from 0 (none) – 10 (very severe), bowel movement	intensity

foods causing symptoms		
food	symptoms	bowel movement

Other: activities, sport, stress, animal contact, smoking, other stress factors

Date: _____   Food-Symptom-Diary

time	Foods, drinks & sweets incl. amount, preparation (raw, steamed, boiled, fried, grilled, rewarmed, peeled), spices and for convenience food ingredients. Medications, vitamin supplements, food supplements, probiotics.	Symptoms	
		type, time, duration, intensity from 0 (none) – 10 (very severe), bowel movement	
			intensity

foods causing symptoms		
food	symptoms	bowel movement

Other: activities, sport, stress, animal contact, smoking, other stress factors

Date: _____   Food-Symptom-Diary

time	Foods, drinks & sweets incl. amount, preparation (raw, steamed, boiled, fried, grilled, rewarmed, peeled), spices and for convenience food ingredients. Medications, vitamin supplements, food supplements, probiotics.	Symptoms	
		type, time, duration, intensity from 0 (none) – 10 (very severe), bowel movement	
			intensity

foods causing symptoms		
food	symptoms	bowel movement

Other: activities, sport, stress, animal contact, smoking, other stress factors

Date: _____   Food-Symptom-Diary

time	Foods, drinks & sweets incl. amount, preparation (raw, steamed, boiled, fried, grilled, rewarmed, peeled), spices and for convenience food ingredients. Medications, vitamin supplements, food supplements, probiotics.	Symptoms	
		type, time, duration, intensity from 0 (none) – 10 (very severe), bowel movement	intensity

foods causing symptoms		
food	symptoms	bowel movement

Other: activities, sport, stress, animal contact, smoking, other stress factors

Date: _____   Food-Symptom-Diary

time	Foods, drinks & sweets incl. amount, preparation (raw, steamed, boiled, fried, grilled, rewarmed, peeled), spices and for convenience food ingredients. Medications, vitamin supplements, food supplements, probiotics.	Symptoms	
		type, time, duration, intensity from 0 (none) – 10 (very severe), bowel movement	intensity

foods causing symptoms		
food	symptoms	bowel movement

Other: activities, sport, stress, animal contact, smoking, other stress factors

Date: _____   Food-Symptom-Diary

time	Foods, drinks & sweets incl. amount, preparation (raw, steamed, boiled, fried, grilled, rewarmed, peeled), spices and for convenience food ingredients. Medications, vitamin supplements, food supplements, probiotics.	Symptoms	
		type, time, duration, intensity from 0 (none) – 10 (very severe), bowel movement	
			intensity

foods causing symptoms		
food	symptoms	bowel movement

Other: activities, sport, stress, animal contact, smoking, other stress factors

Date: _____   Food-Symptom-Diary

time	Foods, drinks & sweets incl. amount, preparation (raw, steamed, boiled, fried, grilled, rewarmed, peeled), spices and for convenience food ingredients. Medications, vitamin supplements, food supplements, probiotics.	Symptoms	
		type, time, duration, intensity from 0 (none) – 10 (very severe), bowel movement	intensity

foods causing symptoms		
food	symptoms	bowel movement

Other: activities, sport, stress, animal contact, smoking, other stress factors

Date: _____   Food-Symptom-Diary

time	Foods, drinks & sweets incl. amount, preparation (raw, steamed, boiled, fried, grilled, rewarmed, peeled), spices and for convenience food ingredients. Medications, vitamin supplements, food supplements, probiotics.	Symptoms	
		type, time, duration, intensity from 0 (none) – 10 (very severe), bowel movement	intensity

foods causing symptoms		
food	symptoms	bowel movement

Other: activities, sport, stress, animal contact, smoking, other stress factors

Date: _____   Food-Symptom-Diary

time	Foods, drinks & sweets incl. amount, preparation (raw, steamed, boiled, fried, grilled, rewarmed, peeled), spices and for convenience food ingredients. Medications, vitamin supplements, food supplements, probiotics.	Symptoms	
		type, time, duration, intensity from 0 (none) – 10 (very severe), bowel movement	intensity

foods causing symptoms		
food	symptoms	bowel movement

Other: activities, sport, stress, animal contact, smoking, other stress factors

Date: _____   Food-Symptom-Diary

time	Foods, drinks & sweets incl. amount, preparation (raw, steamed, boiled, fried, grilled, rewarmed, peeled), spices and for convenience food ingredients. Medications, vitamin supplements, food supplements, probiotics.	Symptoms	
		type, time, duration, intensity from 0 (none) – 10 (very severe), bowel movement	intensity

foods causing symptoms		
food	symptoms	bowel movement

Other: activities, sport, stress, animal contact, smoking, other stress factors

Date: _____   Food-Symptom-Diary

time	Foods, drinks & sweets incl. amount, preparation (raw, steamed, boiled, fried, grilled, rewarmed, peeled), spices and for convenience food ingredients. Medications, vitamin supplements, food supplements, probiotics.	Symptoms	
		type, time, duration, intensity from 0 (none) – 10 (very severe), bowel movement	intensity

foods causing symptoms		
food	symptoms	bowel movement

Other: activities, sport, stress, animal contact, smoking, other stress factors

Date: _____   Food-Symptom-Diary

time	Foods, drinks & sweets incl. amount, preparation (raw, steamed, boiled, fried, grilled, rewarmed, peeled), spices and for convenience food ingredients. Medications, vitamin supplements, food supplements, probiotics.	Symptoms	
		type, time, duration, intensity from 0 (none) – 10 (very severe), bowel movement	intensity

foods causing symptoms		
food	symptoms	bowel movement

Other: activities, sport, stress, animal contact, smoking, other stress factors

Date: _____   Food-Symptom-Diary

time	Foods, drinks & sweets incl. amount, preparation (raw, steamed, boiled, fried, grilled, rewarmed, peeled), spices and for convenience food ingredients. Medications, vitamin supplements, food supplements, probiotics.	Symptoms	
		type, time, duration, intensity from 0 (none) – 10 (very severe), bowel movement	intensity

foods causing symptoms		
food	symptoms	bowel movement

Other: activities, sport, stress, animal contact, smoking, other stress factors

Date: _____ Food-Symptom-Diary

time	Foods, drinks & sweets incl. amount, preparation (raw, steamed, boiled, fried, grilled, rewarmed, peeled), spices and for convenience food ingredients. Medications, vitamin supplements, food supplements, probiotics.	Symptoms	
		type, time, duration, intensity from 0 (none) – 10 (very severe), bowel movement	intensity

foods causing symptoms		
food	symptoms	bowel movement

Other: activities, sport, stress, animal contact, smoking, other stress factors

Date: _____   Food-Symptom-Diary

time	Foods, drinks & sweets incl. amount, preparation (raw, steamed, boiled, fried, grilled, rewarmed, peeled), spices and for convenience food ingredients. Medications, vitamin supplements, food supplements, probiotics.	Symptoms	
		type, time, duration, intensity from 0 (none) – 10 (very severe), bowel movement	
			intensity

foods causing symptoms		
food	symptoms	bowel movement

Other: activities, sport, stress, animal contact, smoking, other stress factors

Date: _____   Food-Symptom-Diary

time	Foods, drinks & sweets incl. amount, preparation (raw, steamed, boiled, fried, grilled, rewarmed, peeled), spices and for convenience food ingredients. Medications, vitamin supplements, food supplements, probiotics.	Symptoms	
		type, time, duration, intensity from 0 (none) – 10 (very severe), bowel movement	
			intensity

foods causing symptoms		
food	symptoms	bowel movement

Other: activities, sport, stress, animal contact, smoking, other stress factors

Date: _____   Food-Symptom-Diary

time	Foods, drinks & sweets incl. amount, preparation (raw, steamed, boiled, fried, grilled, rewarmed, peeled), spices and for convenience food ingredients. Medications, vitamin supplements, food supplements, probiotics.	Symptoms	
		type, time, duration, intensity from 0 (none) – 10 (very severe), bowel movement	intensity

foods causing symptoms		
food	symptoms	bowel movement

Other: activities, sport, stress, animal contact, smoking, other stress factors

Date: _____   Food-Symptom-Diary

time	Foods, drinks & sweets incl. amount, preparation (raw, steamed, boiled, fried, grilled, rewarmed, peeled), spices and for convenience food ingredients. Medications, vitamin supplements, food supplements, probiotics.	Symptoms	
		type, time, duration, intensity from 0 (none) – 10 (very severe), bowel movement	
			intensity

foods causing symptoms		
food	symptoms	bowel movement

Other: activities, sport, stress, animal contact, smoking, other stress factors

Date: _____   Food-Symptom-Diary

time	Foods, drinks & sweets incl. amount, preparation (raw, steamed, boiled, fried, grilled, rewarmed, peeled), spices and for convenience food ingredients. Medications, vitamin supplements, food supplements, probiotics.	Symptoms	
		type, time, duration, intensity from 0 (none) – 10 (very severe), bowel movement	intensity

foods causing symptoms		
food	symptoms	bowel movement

Other: activities, sport, stress, animal contact, smoking, other stress factors

Date: _____   Food-Symptom-Diary

time	Foods, drinks & sweets incl. amount, preparation (raw, steamed, boiled, fried, grilled, rewarmed, peeled), spices and for convenience food ingredients. Medications, vitamin supplements, food supplements, probiotics.	Symptoms	
		type, time, duration, intensity from 0 (none) – 10 (very severe), bowel movement	
			intensity

foods causing symptoms		
food	symptoms	bowel movement

Other: activities, sport, stress, animal contact, smoking, other stress factors

Date: _____   Food-Symptom-Diary

time	Foods, drinks & sweets incl. amount, preparation (raw, steamed, boiled, fried, grilled, rewarmed, peeled), spices and for convenience food ingredients. Medications, vitamin supplements, food supplements, probiotics.	Symptoms	
		type, time, duration, intensity from 0 (none) – 10 (very severe), bowel movement	intensity

foods causing symptoms		
food	symptoms	bowel movement

Other: activities, sport, stress, animal contact, smoking, other stress factors

Date: _____   Food-Symptom-Diary

time	Foods, drinks & sweets incl. amount, preparation (raw, steamed, boiled, fried, grilled, rewarmed, peeled), spices and for convenience food ingredients. Medications, vitamin supplements, food supplements, probiotics.	Symptoms	
		type, time, duration, intensity from 0 (none) – 10 (very severe), bowel movement	
			intensity

foods causing symptoms		
food	symptoms	bowel movement

Other: activities, sport, stress, animal contact, smoking, other stress factors

Date: _____   Food-Symptom-Diary

time	Foods, drinks & sweets incl. amount, preparation (raw, steamed, boiled, fried, grilled, rewarmed, peeled), spices and for convenience food ingredients. Medications, vitamin supplements, food supplements, probiotics.	Symptoms	
		type, time, duration, intensity from 0 (none) – 10 (very severe), bowel movement	
			intensity

foods causing symptoms		
food	symptoms	bowel movement

Other: activities, sport, stress, animal contact, smoking, other stress factors

Date: _____   Food-Symptom-Diary

time	Foods, drinks & sweets incl. amount, preparation (raw, steamed, boiled, fried, grilled, rewarmed, peeled), spices and for convenience food ingredients. Medications, vitamin supplements, food supplements, probiotics.	Symptoms	
		type, time, duration, intensity from 0 (none) – 10 (very severe), bowel movement	intensity

foods causing symptoms		
food	symptoms	bowel movement

Other: activities, sport, stress, animal contact, smoking, other stress factors

Date: _____   Food-Symptom-Diary

time	Foods, drinks & sweets incl. amount, preparation (raw, steamed, boiled, fried, grilled, rewarmed, peeled), spices and for convenience food ingredients. Medications, vitamin supplements, food supplements, probiotics.	Symptoms	
		type, time, duration, intensity from 0 (none) – 10 (very severe), bowel movement	intensity

foods causing symptoms		
food	symptoms	bowel movement

Other: activities, sport, stress, animal contact, smoking, other stress factors

Date: _____   Food-Symptom-Diary

time	Foods, drinks & sweets incl. amount, preparation (raw, steamed, boiled, fried, grilled, rewarmed, peeled), spices and for convenience food ingredients. Medications, vitamin supplements, food supplements, probiotics.	Symptoms	
		type, time, duration, intensity from 0 (none) – 10 (very severe), bowel movement	intensity

foods causing symptoms		
food	symptoms	bowel movement

Other: activities, sport, stress, animal contact, smoking, other stress factors

Date: _____ Food-Symptom-Diary

time	Foods, drinks & sweets incl. amount, preparation (raw, steamed, boiled, fried, grilled, rewarmed, peeled), spices and for convenience food ingredients. Medications, vitamin supplements, food supplements, probiotics.	Symptoms	
		type, time, duration, intensity from 0 (none) – 10 (very severe), bowel movement	
			intensity

foods causing symptoms		
food	symptoms	bowel movement

Other: activities, sport, stress, animal contact, smoking, other stress factors

Date: _____   Food-Symptom-Diary

time	Foods, drinks & sweets incl. amount, preparation (raw, steamed, boiled, fried, grilled, rewarmed, peeled), spices and for convenience food ingredients. Medications, vitamin supplements, food supplements, probiotics.	Symptoms	
		type, time, duration, intensity from 0 (none) – 10 (very severe), bowel movement	intensity

foods causing symptoms		
food	symptoms	bowel movement

Other: activities, sport, stress, animal contact, smoking, other stress factors

Date: _____   Food-Symptom-Diary

time	Foods, drinks & sweets incl. amount, preparation (raw, steamed, boiled, fried, grilled, rewarmed, peeled), spices and for convenience food ingredients. Medications, vitamin supplements, food supplements, probiotics.	Symptoms	
		type, time, duration, intensity from 0 (none) – 10 (very severe), bowel movement	
			intensity

foods causing symptoms		
food	symptoms	bowel movement

Other: activities, sport, stress, animal contact, smoking, other stress factors

Date: _____   Food-Symptom-Diary

time	Foods, drinks & sweets incl. amount, preparation (raw, steamed, boiled, fried, grilled, rewarmed, peeled), spices and for convenience food ingredients. Medications, vitamin supplements, food supplements, probiotics.	Symptoms	
		type, time, duration, intensity from 0 (none) – 10 (very severe), bowel movement	intensity

foods causing symptoms		
food	symptoms	bowel movement

Other: activities, sport, stress, animal contact, smoking, other stress factors

Date: _____   Food-Symptom-Diary

time	Foods, drinks & sweets incl. amount, preparation (raw, steamed, boiled, fried, grilled, rewarmed, peeled), spices and for convenience food ingredients. Medications, vitamin supplements, food supplements, probiotics.	Symptoms	
		type, time, duration, intensity from 0 (none) – 10 (very severe), bowel movement	
			intensity

foods causing symptoms		
food	symptoms	bowel movement

Other: activities, sport, stress, animal contact, smoking, other stress factors

Date: _____   Food-Symptom-Diary

time	Foods, drinks & sweets incl. amount, preparation (raw, steamed, boiled, fried, grilled, rewarmed, peeled), spices and for convenience food ingredients. Medications, vitamin supplements, food supplements, probiotics.	Symptoms	
		type, time, duration, intensity from 0 (none) – 10 (very severe), bowel movement	intensity

foods causing symptoms		
food	symptoms	bowel movement

Other: activities, sport, stress, animal contact, smoking, other stress factors

Date: _____   Food-Symptom-Diary

time	Foods, drinks & sweets incl. amount, preparation (raw, steamed, boiled, fried, grilled, rewarmed, peeled), spices and for convenience food ingredients. Medications, vitamin supplements, food supplements, probiotics.	Symptoms	
		type, time, duration, intensity from 0 (none) – 10 (very severe), bowel movement	
			intensity

foods causing symptoms		
food	symptoms	bowel movement

Other: activities, sport, stress, animal contact, smoking, other stress factors

Date: _____ Food-Symptom-Diary

time	Foods, drinks & sweets incl. amount, preparation (raw, steamed, boiled, fried, grilled, rewarmed, peeled), spices and for convenience food ingredients. Medications, vitamin supplements, food supplements, probiotics.	Symptoms	
		type, time, duration, intensity from 0 (none) – 10 (very severe), bowel movement	
			intensity

foods causing symptoms		
food	symptoms	bowel movement

Other: activities, sport, stress, animal contact, smoking, other stress factors

Date: _____   Food-Symptom-Diary

time	Foods, drinks & sweets incl. amount, preparation (raw, steamed, boiled, fried, grilled, rewarmed, peeled), spices and for convenience food ingredients. Medications, vitamin supplements, food supplements, probiotics.	Symptoms	
		type, time, duration, intensity from 0 (none) – 10 (very severe), bowel movement	
			intensity

foods causing symptoms		
food	symptoms	bowel movement

Other: activities, sport, stress, animal contact, smoking, other stress factors

Date: _____   Food-Symptom-Diary

time	Foods, drinks & sweets incl. amount, preparation (raw, steamed, boiled, fried, grilled, rewarmed, peeled), spices and for convenience food ingredients. Medications, vitamin supplements, food supplements, probiotics.	Symptoms	
		type, time, duration, intensity from 0 (none) – 10 (very severe), bowel movement	intensity

foods causing symptoms		
food	symptoms	bowel movement

Other: activities, sport, stress, animal contact, smoking, other stress factors

Date: _____   Food-Symptom-Diary

time	Foods, drinks & sweets incl. amount, preparation (raw, steamed, boiled, fried, grilled, rewarmed, peeled), spices and for convenience food ingredients. Medications, vitamin supplements, food supplements, probiotics.	Symptoms	
		type, time, duration, intensity from 0 (none) – 10 (very severe), bowel movement	
			intensity

foods causing symptoms		
food	symptoms	bowel movement

Other: activities, sport, stress, animal contact, smoking, other stress factors

Date: _____   Food-Symptom-Diary

time	Foods, drinks & sweets incl. amount, preparation (raw, steamed, boiled, fried, grilled, rewarmed, peeled), spices and for convenience food ingredients. Medications, vitamin supplements, food supplements, probiotics.	Symptoms	
		type, time, duration, intensity from 0 (none) – 10 (very severe), bowel movement	
			intensity

foods causing symptoms		
food	symptoms	bowel movement

Other: activities, sport, stress, animal contact, smoking, other stress factors

Date: _____   Food-Symptom-Diary

time	Foods, drinks & sweets incl. amount, preparation (raw, steamed, boiled, fried, grilled, rewarmed, peeled), spices and for convenience food ingredients. Medications, vitamin supplements, food supplements, probiotics.	Symptoms	
		type, time, duration, intensity from 0 (none) – 10 (very severe), bowel movement	
			intensity

foods causing symptoms		
food	symptoms	bowel movement

Other: activities, sport, stress, animal contact, smoking, other stress factors

Date: _____   Food-Symptom-Diary

time	Foods, drinks & sweets incl. amount, preparation (raw, steamed, boiled, fried, grilled, rewarmed, peeled), spices and for convenience food ingredients. Medications, vitamin supplements, food supplements, probiotics.	Symptoms	
		type, time, duration, intensity from 0 (none) – 10 (very severe), bowel movement	intensity

foods causing symptoms		
food	symptoms	bowel movement

Other: activities, sport, stress, animal contact, smoking, other stress factors

Date: _____ Food-Symptom-Diary

time	Foods, drinks & sweets incl. amount, preparation (raw, steamed, boiled, fried, grilled, rewarmed, peeled), spices and for convenience food ingredients. Medications, vitamin supplements, food supplements, probiotics.	Symptoms	
		type, time, duration, intensity from 0 (none) – 10 (very severe), bowel movement	
			intensity

foods causing symptoms		
food	symptoms	bowel movement

Other: activities, sport, stress, animal contact, smoking, other stress factors

Date: _____   Food-Symptom-Diary

time	Foods, drinks & sweets incl. amount, preparation (raw, steamed, boiled, fried, grilled, rewarmed, peeled), spices and for convenience food ingredients. Medications, vitamin supplements, food supplements, probiotics.	Symptoms	
		type, time, duration, intensity from 0 (none) – 10 (very severe), bowel movement	intensity

foods causing symptoms		
food	symptoms	bowel movement

Other: activities, sport, stress, animal contact, smoking, other stress factors

Date: _____   Food-Symptom-Diary

time	Foods, drinks & sweets incl. amount, preparation (raw, steamed, boiled, fried, grilled, rewarmed, peeled), spices and for convenience food ingredients. Medications, vitamin supplements, food supplements, probiotics.	Symptoms	
		type, time, duration, intensity from 0 (none) – 10 (very severe), bowel movement	
			intensity

foods causing symptoms		
food	symptoms	bowel movement

Other: activities, sport, stress, animal contact, smoking, other stress factors

Date: _____   Food-Symptom-Diary

time	Foods, drinks & sweets incl. amount, preparation (raw, steamed, boiled, fried, grilled, rewarmed, peeled), spices and for convenience food ingredients. Medications, vitamin supplements, food supplements, probiotics.	Symptoms	
		type, time, duration, intensity from 0 (none) – 10 (very severe), bowel movement	intensity

foods causing symptoms		
food	symptoms	bowel movement

Other: activities, sport, stress, animal contact, smoking, other stress factors

Foods & drinks, well tolerated

In this table you may list foods & drinks incl. amount, preparation (raw, steamed, boiled, fried, grilled, rewarmed, peeled), spices and for convenience food ingredients. Medications, vitamin supplements, food supplements, probiotics, that are <u>well tolerated</u>.

Date	foods & drinks	amount
1.1.	black tea with milk	200 ml
1.1.	yoghurt 150 g (brand name)	150 g
1.1.	strawberry yam (brand name)	1 teaspoon
1.1.	bread (whole-grain)	1 slice
1.1.	salami	25 g
1.1.	carrots, steamed	200 g
1.1.	probiotic (brand name)	2 capsules
1.1.	tomato	~ 100 g
1.1.	mozzarella	~ 100 g
1.1.	cucumber, peeled	100 g

Foods & drinks, <u>well tolerated</u>

Date	foods & drinks	amount

Foods & drinks, <u>well tolerated</u>

Date	foods & drinks	amount

Foods & drinks, <u>well tolerated</u>

Date	foods & drinks	amount

Foods & drinks, causing symptoms

In this table you may list foods & drinks incl. amount, preparation (raw, steamed, boiled, fried, grilled, rewarmed, peeled), spices and for convenience food ingredients. Medications, vitamin supplements, food supplements, probiotics, that are well tolerated.

Date	foods & drinks	amount
1.1.	Beer (dark)(brand name)	½ L
1.1.	chewing gum (brand name, contains sorbitol and isomaltol)	3 pieces

Foods & drinks, causing symptoms

Date	foods & drinks	amount

Foods & drinks, causing symptoms

Date	foods & drinks	amount

Foods & drinks, causing symptoms

Date	foods & drinks	amount

Foods & drinks, alternately well or badly tolerated

In this table you may list foods & drinks incl. amount, preparation (raw, steamed, boiled, fried, grilled, rewarmed, peeled), spices and for convenience food ingredients. Medications, vitamin supplements, food supplements, probiotics, that are <u>alternately well or badly tolerated</u>.

Date	foods & drinks	amount

Foods & drinks, alternately well or badly tolerated

Date	foods & drinks	amount

Foods & drinks, alternately well or badly tolerated

Date	foods & drinks	amount

Foods & drinks, alternately well or badly tolerated

Date	foods & drinks	amount

Lists of foods, with high predictive value for specific food intolerances

The following lists are not complete lists of foods to be avoided in the context of various intolerances. These lists rather name foods that are highly indicative for different food intolerances since these foods frequently cause symptoms if the respective intolerance is underlying. Therefore these lists are very helpful in tracking down individual food intolerances.

Lactose

Foods badly tolerated with lactose-intolerance:

product	lactose content per 100 g	possible test meal
concentrated milk	55-60 g	2 tablespoons
soured milk	14 g	150 g
whole milk chocolate	9-11 g	1 bar
processed cheese	6-7 g	100 g
ice cream	6-9 g	150 g
unskimmed milk	5 g	2 cups
whey	5 g	2 cups

Fructose

Foods badly tolerated with fructose-intolerance:

product	fructose content per 100 g	possible test meal
diabetic chocolate	50-55 g	1 bar
honey	36-40 g	50 g
raisin	34 g	100 g
apple, dried	34 g	100 g
quince jelly	18 g	50 g
Italian plum, dried	12 g	100 g
applesauce	7,5 g	50 g
apple juice	7 g	2 glasses

Sorbitol

Foods badly tolerated with sorbitol-intolerance:

product	sorbitol content per 100 g	possible test meal
diabetic sweets	up to 95 g	50 g
diabetic jam	up to 11 g	25 g
pear, dried	11 g	50 g
plum butter	6 g	100 g
chewing gum (sorbitol)	variable	5 – 10 pieces
mint-sweets		
apricot, dried	5 g	100 g
apple, dried	3,5 g	150 g

Trehalose

Foods badly tolerated with trehalose-intolerance:

high trehalose content
mushrooms

Fructans / Fructooligosaccharides / FOS

Foods badly tolerated with fructan/fructooligosaccharide-intolerance:

high fructan/fructooligosaccharide content
bread, pasta, cereals, chicory coffee
peach, kaki, nectarine, water melon
cashew nut, chickpeas, lentils, Jerusalem artichoke
inulin, oligofructose

Galactans / Galactooligosaccharides / GOS

Foods badly tolerated with galactan/galactooligosaccharide-intolerance:

high galactan/galactooligosaccharide content
beans, chickpeas, lentils

Gluten

Foods badly tolerated with gluten/wheat-intolerance:

high gluten content
baguette, bun/roll light, ciabatta, white bread
wheat bread, wheat toast, wheat pasta
wheat beer

Histamine

The food histamine content is very variable and depends on the freshness of the foods. With an underlying histamine-intolerance foods with a high histamine content or foods that facilitate endogenous histamine release (so called histamine-liberators) may cause symptoms:

high histamine content	histamine-liberators
tuna	pineapple
beer (top-fermented, wheat beer)	tomato
red wine, sparkling wine	chocolate, cocoa
camembert-cheese, brie-cheese	citrus fruits
balsamic vinegar	kiwi
sauerkraut	seafood
anchovy	glutamate
	strawberry

Salicylates

The food salicylate content is variable. Foods badly tolerated with salicylate-intolerance:

high salicylate content
dried fruits
apple – apricot - strawberry – currant – citrus fruits
white mushroom – bell pepper - tomato
almonds
licorice
sausages and cold meat
yeast extract (marmite), mustard
aspirin

Biogenic Amines

Biogenic amines develop during food maturation from proteins and their content in food is very variable. In principle, the more mature the food, the higher the content of biogenic amines, the fresher the food, the lower the content of biogenic amines. Foods often badly tolerated with an intolerance to biogenic amines are:

high content of biogenic amines
cheese
wine, beer
chocolate
pineapple – banana – orange
soy
yeast extract (marmite)
meat products
tomato, ketchup
nuts
sauerkraut

Pseudoallergens (Mast Cells)

Pseudoallergens are substances which induce a release of messengers from innate defense cells (mast cells) and thereby cause allergy-like symptoms. Since most pseudoallergens are food additives it is important to watch out for food additives. Persons with sensitivity to pseudoallergens poorly tolerate the following:

pseudoallergens	included in:
preservatives E200-E299 and E1105	almost all industrially manufactured foods
emulsifiers E322, E400- E495	sauces, salad dressings
acidity regulators E300-E385	almost all industrially manufactured foods
food colors, E 100-E180	many industrially manufactured foods
lectins	beans (especially raw)
sulfites, E150 and E220-E228	wine, dried fruit, chips, dried meat/fish products

E-numbers for European food labelling

„Wisdom of Crowds"

Some foods cause symptoms for unknown reasons. The following list names foods that cause symptoms in more than 15% of people.

Symptoms in more than x percent	foods
> 30%	cabbage, beans, legume, strongly spiced food, fried
> 20%	fat foods, fried foods, onions, cucumber salad, carbonated drinks
> 15%	coffee, nuts, orange juice, milk, cheese, bell peppers, sauerkraut

Made in the USA
San Bernardino, CA
31 January 2019